This is a true story.

(a shit one)

Introduction 1
Finding out 5
Chemotherapy 23
Surgery 61
Radiotherapy 91
The End 109
Acknowledgements 113

Introduction

I am a soldier. I joined the Army as an Officer in the Parachute Regiment before transferring to the Army Air Corps and becoming an Apache Attack Helicopter Pilot. This means I have been trained to be resilient. Trained to cope with stress. Trained to remain optimistic and focussed when confronted with the most significant of challenges. My Regimental moto is Utrinque Paratus; Ready for Anything. But, on the 25 October 2023, I was not ready. I was more scared than I've ever been in my entire life. That was the day we found out Alex had breast cancer.

At the time we had just celebrated our ninth wedding anniversary, and our daughters were aged 1 and 4.

This book is a chronological account of my feelings as we journeyed along the helter-skelter, roller-coaster ride that dealing with cancer is.

Starting from the day Alex was diagnosed, I decided to keep a journal. Some days included a lot of detail, others just a couple of words. Initially I wanted to ensure I was recording the important information in case Alex asked me a question about something the medical staff had told us. It quickly became apparent that I was using it as an outlet for my feelings and that it would be a good way for me to monitor my ups and downs.

What follows is a summary of the feelings I felt at each stage, with some entries from the diary being copied verbatim and discussed now that some time has passed. Other entries will remain private forever, I don't need to fall out with friends and family for comments I wrote in the heat of the moment! In another attempt to protect those I love the most, I have used fake names for everyone I talk about.

I hope that this book can raise awareness, help people in similar situations, and raise money for the fantastic charities who supported us through the shittest experience of my life.

If you're a dad or partner in a similar situation to me, I hope this book can give you some sense that you're not alone. It is crap, but you will get through it.

If you're the one with cancer, a family member, a friend, or colleague of someone you know in a similar situation, I hope this book offers a glimpse into how that person may be feeling and can be used as a conversation starter to see how they are. I found the hardest thing was starting the conversation, especially with those I wanted to talk to the most. Communication is a two-way process. It's easy to forget that when you think nobody is talking to you.

Finding out

Alex had a lump on her breast that had previously been checked by a GP. Over time it started to grow and become uncomfortable. She complained about it a few times and I said she should go and have it checked out. It took a few weeks, but she eventually did. The GP decided it needed further investigation and sent her for an ultrasound and biopsy.

It's worth noting early on that throughout the period this book covers, we were based at a camp that was four-to-five hours drive away from our nearest family. We were, however, fortunate to have some excellent friends who lived nearby and family that would frequently make the journey and stay with us to help out.

The story starts the day before we got the results from the biopsy. My parents had come to look after the girls, and the day before the appointment I went for a walk with my dad. It's the first entry I wrote in the diary:

24 October. Tuesday.

Mum and dad have come to look after the girls for the appointment tomorrow. Went on a dog walk with dad. We chatted but not about tomorrow. I said I'm nervous. I think he understood it meant I was scared.

Looking back now, this was the first time I wanted to talk more but couldn't. My dad has been the main male role model throughout my life; and he's been a great one. But, despite having open and frank conversations about all sorts of things over the years, when it came to this, I just couldn't find a way to explain how I was feeling. I guess I didn't want to admit the fact I was shitting myself, as it could have all been about nothing and I wanted to look cool and calm under pressure.

The next extract is from the day we got told the results of the biopsy (spoiler alert – the news wasn't good news; this book would be pretty short if it was! It would be a pretty rubbish story even by my standards).

25 October. Wednesday.

The day we got told. I held Alex's hand as much as I could. I didn't shake hands with the doctor or nurse. Probably should have done. They had a difficult job, and I didn't say thank you. Good manners cost nothing, and dignity will help us through this. Alex said she knew from the moment the nurse called her name to go into the room. The doctor reassured us it wasn't the same lump as a couple of years ago, not sure about that.

My stomach hurts and I just wanted to cry. The drive home was long, and we got stuck in traffic.

We are due to visit family and stay at my parents for the weekend. We decided to try and still go. I loaded the car. So stressed, just threw everything in. I kept mum and dad at arm's length. Didn't want to talk to them.

Finally made it to their house after a 5-hour drive. I unpacked the car and went to bed. Sobbed and sobbed as soon as I was on my own.

Alex slept in a different room with Sophie, and I have Charlotte with me. Charlotte needs to go cold-turkey from breast feeding, which'll be shit.

Sophie, our eldest daughter, was 4 at the time and Charlotte was just 13-months old.

Looking back now, I was a mess for the first few days. My mind was scrambled, and I could not think straight. I'm slightly proud that I realised I needed to be grateful for the doctors and nurses, but also ashamed that my entire focus wasn't on Alex.

To show how much of a mess I was, take a look at what I wrote the next day:

26 October. Thursday.

Went for a run after breakfast. Pulled my hood over my head and cried and cried whilst I ran. Started saying to myself out loud: "Alex has cancer" "It is far from ideal" "It's going to be tough" "We will do it together" "I am a good dad". Sobbed. Repeated those words over and over again.

Can you imagine what I looked like to the people I ran past who were just trying to have a nice morning dog walk! Snot and tears and reciting phrases like a mad man! Luckily, I don't think I bumped into anyone I knew.

I think this was the first indication of some of my training kicking in. I think I subconsciously knew I was going to have to talk to people about it, but I also knew my emotions wouldn't let me hold a conversation about it for very long. By reciting those words like a mantra, I was able to get to the point where they simply rolled off my tongue. The phrase "It's far from ideal" added humour to the conversation and made it easier to talk about. I was rehearsing something I knew would be difficult to do.

The next day, 27 October, I took Charlotte and Sophie to my sister's (Rose's) house to give Alex some space to process it all. I was alone in Rose's kitchen, and she asked how I was. The bloody rehearsals didn't work and when I opened my mouth to speak I just started crying. Fucking sisters. This was the first time I'd outwardly shown emotion in front of someone. She gave me a hug.

From the outset I knew my role was to be the strong and supportive father and husband. I knew I needed to process my emotions, but was also acutely aware that it wouldn't do much good for Alex, and especially the girls, to see me crying. It was a continual balancing act to manage my emotions, let Alex know I cared, and maintain as much 'normality' as I could for the girls.

The next day was Saturday, and I started my stint as a low-level gambling addict. Over the next few weeks and months, I recall in the diary how many lottery tickets I purchased. The idea was that somehow winning a shedload of cash would make the situation better. Clearly, becoming a multi-millionaire overnight would have probably screwed with our minds in an incredibly unhelpful way at that moment! But, anyhow, for the next few months I'd happily drop 40 or 50 quid on a load of lucky dips in the belief that it might be the solution to our problems. Idiot.

After a few days we decided to go home. On the way we stopped to see Alex's family and friends.

29 October. Sunday

Decided to drive home. Called in at Alex's Dad's house. Sophie playing up a bit but enjoyed seeing Alex's old bedroom.

Went to the park to meet up with Alex's friends. Alex cried as soon as she saw Claire. Sophie knew.

This is the first time I note Sophie's astuteness about the situation. Kids aren't stupid. They notice way more than we give them credit for. When Alex was crying with her friends I took the girls off to one side. They were happy enough, but Sophie asked me why Mummy was crying. I explained how she was sad because she was poorly. We had decided to be honest with Sophie as much as possible. Alex explained to her about the lump in her breast being 'cancer' and that she will need lots of medicine to get better. It never got any easier, but I think it was the right approach.

Luckily, our local Macmillan centre had loads of books about helping children cope when their parents have cancer. It was, however, still a bit of a challenge to find the right books that were applicable to us. We had caught

Alex's cancer relatively early so some of the books that talked about death were certainly not wanted, but there were many others that explained things like hair-loss, fatigue, and surgery which offered invaluable advice and insights.

When we got home, we rearranged the bedrooms. I had Charlotte in with me and Alex was in with Sophie. It was to help Charlotte cope with suddenly being forced onto solid foods and no more breast milk. If she could smell or sense Alex in the night, then that's all she would want. When it was just me and my hairy chest she settled surprisingly quickly. Poor Charlotte.

The next day wasn't one of my finest moments.

31 October. Tuesday.

Literally shit myself. We'd gone shopping and I went to do a little fart. Ended up doing a shart. Not a big one, just a bit of wetness between my cheeks. Hopefully it's just something I ate. Didn't tell Alex, just gave her the girls and quicky ran to the toilet.

It's Halloween tonight. Took the girls trick-or-treating and saw loads of people we know. It's hard to explain my feelings. I am scared and angry. So angry.

Alex's mind is all over the place. She is really worried. She is a little forgetful and gets annoyed with me if I ask her to make a decision or clarify anything. Her mind must be going a million miles per hour.

There are a few things to digest (or not) from this extract. Firstly, it's the first time I acknowledge a physical manifestation of the stress I was under. During this journey I have had regular outbreaks of spots, my digestive system has frequently been unhappy, and my hair line has receded. Sure, some of these things may not have been directly attributable to dealing with the stress of Alex having cancer, but they probably were to some extent.

I realised early on I needed to look after my physical wellbeing in order to maintain my psychological wellbeing.

1 November. Wednesday.

In the gym. Feels good.

I'm hurting and scared about the future. Never felt like this before. Want to talk to someone.

I think this was me telling myself to reach out more. I have some great mates who have been with me along every step of this journey. Some I've known since primary school, others from university, and some from work. There's nothing better than having a good friend. The one who answers your call or texts back. Sometimes they reach out first, sometimes they listen, sometimes they can say just the right thing. I hope I can be as a good mate in the future to those who have been there for me throughout this. I've found the most telling sign of a good friend is that they don't judge you when you're venting. It's important to vent when you are stressed.

The diary was a good place to vent. It was a safe place to vent. I often wrote things in the diary and then decided to talk to a real person. It was a good filter to make sure I knew what I wanted to say and who I wanted to say it to.

3 November. Friday.

Worst week of my life. Boiler broke, pet insurance due, car broken (I smashed the headlight against a pheasant)*, Alex has cancer.*

I'm telling myself that it'll get worse as motivation.

How uplifting. I was telling myself that life was going to get shitter in an attempt to enjoy the present moment, which was shit.

Over the next few days things continued to be hard. Charlotte started teething and was awake every 40 minutes through the night. We were still sleeping separately so I dealt with that on my own. Alex's stress and anxiety continued to rise. I wanted to take the girls out a couple of times, but Alex wanted to stay home so we did. It's a difficult balancing act, but you do what you think is right in the moment.

On the 6 November Alex had an MRI scan. She was becoming convinced the cancer had spread. She said the nurse gave her a funny (pitying) look on the way out of the scan. I found myself reassuring her that if it had spread then we would deal with it. This was the first time I had to stop myself just saying wishful things.

There is no point in denying what is happening. Positivity and wishful thinking are great, but don't get mentioned much in medical journals. I decided to focus on confidence. I tried to give Alex the confidence that whatever happened, we would be able to deal with it.

7 November. Tuesday.

Went into work. It's nice to deal with things that don't really matter. Took life insurance out for me.

I'm lucky to have a job that I love doing, colleagues that I like spending time with, and managers who gave me all the time and space I needed.

Work was a sanctuary for me. I needed to escape the house. I needed to feel like I had a purpose beyond being a husband and dad. A regular dose of normality was very helpful for me throughout the journey.

Unbeknownst to Alex, I had looked into our life insurance policies and realised we didn't have enough cover! I thought I'd be ok if Alex did die as I earned the majority of our income, but I was really scared that if *I* randomly died that she wouldn't have enough to be comfortable! I hid the fact I took an extra policy out from her as I didn't want her to know I was thinking about death as a possibility. And the last thing she needed was to start thinking about me dying!

8 November. Wednesday.

MRI scan results showed swollen lymph nodes. Both me and Alex are scared.

I went to get my flu jab and broke down crying when the nurse asked me how I was. That was embarrassing.

This was one of the 'bad days'. When you get bad results you think the worst. Even though swollen lymph nodes can just be a sign of your body fighting an infection, we both took it to mean the cancer was spreading. It was terrifying. I found myself constantly thinking about 'What if'. What if it's spread? What if she dies? What if she dies quickly? What if she dies slowly?

The unknown is bad, the imagined is worse.

Having a mini break-down in front of the nurse didn't help. I'd been trying to remain strong for Alex and be confident about the future. Then I got asked by a stranger if I'm OK and turned into a mess. Felt pathetic. As you'd expect, the nurse was brilliant. She let me cry, offered support and talked me round. A couple days later I got the phone call I was expecting from the doctor asking if I was OK, the nurse had left a note on the computer about what had happened. It felt good to know the system was there to support me if I needed it.

The following days continued to be hard. Alex got sent for a mammogram and more biopsies. At one point they thought it may have spread to her abdomen and pelvis so booked her a full-body CT scan. The appointment was made for 2-weeks' time. The wait was going to be hell.

On 9 November (Thursday) I found Alex crying and gave her a cuddle. She sobbed saying "please please

please". She was praying that it hadn't spread. That was hard to deal with.

They pushed Alex to the front of the queue for a CT scan so we only had to wait a couple of days in the end, which was good. We both appreciated the appointment coming earlier, but it was bittersweet as we realised it was because her case must be serious. Luckily, we got the results the next day and it hadn't spread.

10 November. Friday.

Alex was crying and explained to Sophie what was going on with the cancer. Sophie listened and then ran off. She went and got a pen and paper and drew a picture of the two of them smiling and surrounded by love hearts. Struggled to hold back the tears myself!

As if it wasn't hard enough, Sophie went and did things like that. I love that girl!

11 November. Saturday.

Alex felt good enough to be left with the girls so I went for a haircut. I decided I didn't want to talk about the cancer with the hairdresser. The hairdresser asked me a completely innocent question about Alex and the girls. I welled up and couldn't talk. We changed the subject in time, but it was really hard. If I'd just told her about it, I reckon I would've been fine.

I had actually got pretty good at talking to people about what was going on (probably thanks to my crazy mantra chanting runs). But on this occasion I tried to hide from reality. It was a good lesson for me in acceptance. It is a lot easier to deal with a shit situation if you accept it as such. I'm sure there's probably some very good scientific studies on suppression, but I know from experience it doesn't work and it doesn't help. I remember feeling so embarrassed about crying in the barbershop. There were a few other people in there who probably hadn't heard the conversation but definitely saw me cry a little. On a positive note, I'm glad I realised my mistake and knew what to differently the next time.

12 November. Sunday.

Work has been really good and very supportive. Chris (my boss) *has been great. I'm struggling to feel like a good husband because I still want to work, not because I want to progress but because I don't want to feel like a sponger, or feel vulnerable. I think it is hard for me to accept help. But I need it.*

We asked our friend Emma to take some photos of us as a family before Alex starts chemotherapy tomorrow.

Feeling vulnerable is an incredibly difficult emotion for me. I think wanting to work feeds directly into this. By accepting I could not perform at work was accepting I wasn't superhuman. But I'm not superhuman. It is easy to say there is a need to prioritise differently when faced with significant life events, but re-prioritising isn't easy. If something was a priority before the event, it's because it held some form of value to you. That value will still exist, even though something becomes even more important. With time, re-prioritising did eventually become easier to do and accept.

It was Alex's idea to have some photos as a family before chemotherapy started. It was a great idea. Tinged with sadness but I love the pictures we got and will cherish them forever.

So; we've been given the bad news. Felt guilty about not being nicer to the doctors and nurses. Ran like a mental-asylum escapee. Shit myself. Helped Charlotte go cold-turkey from breast feeding. Sobbed; on my own, with family, and with strangers. Thought it's spread and been told it hadn't. Been amazed at the astuteness, and cuteness, of Sophie. And realised I'm not very good at being vulnerable. Seems like a lot, and we hadn't even started treatment yet!

Chemotherapy

13 November. Monday.

Chemotherapy day 1. So surreal. Just kind of on a weird autopilot. Everything feels so normal and calm. The team at the hospital are great. I need to remember the details about Alex's medication:

Dexamethasone. 3 tablets at breakfast with food, for 3 days.

Fluconazole. From day 8 take 1 tablet at breakfast for a week.

Ondansetron. Anti-sickness. 1 tablet twice a day for 3 days starting tomorrow.

Metoclopramide. Anti-sickness. 2 tablets up to 3 times a day as required.

Steroid injection. Everyday at 6pm for 1 week. Pinch, jab at 45°, inject. Keep it in the fridge.

That was a heavy day. We both approached it in a very matter-of-fact way. You can see that from how I made notes about the medication. It was a to-do list with minimal emotion. I probably wasn't capable of processing my emotions at the time. I remember feeling happy that we were starting the treatment, and grateful for the NHS.

The steroid injection was probably the worst bit for me. I injected Alex every day for a week after each dose of chemotherapy. We tried to hide it from the girls, but obviously couldn't hide from it myself! It makes the illness incredibly real when you have to prepare a syringe and then inject the person you love with a medicine you hope is working.

15 November. Wednesday.

Sophie cried at the school drop-off. She told Alex she is sad that she is poorly but will be happy when she is better.

It's moments like that which hurt the most. I have no idea how much Sophie understood about what was going on, but I know it was more than I thought. I hate that she was suffering. I remember reading everything I could about how to help children with parents who have cancer. I saw it as important as remaining strong for Alex.

Over the next few entries in the diary, I talked about fatigue starting to kick in and the fact I was still dreaming of winning the lottery. With hindsight, it amuses me to see myself writing about fatigue; it was nothing compared to what would come.

A sad thing happened on the 18 November that I can still remember vividly now. I was taking Charlotte for a swimming lesson and as I went to put her in the car seat, Alex made a comment that I'd put Charlotte in a coat rather than a jumper and she would be too hot. I snapped. I shouted and swore at Alex. She had done nothing wrong, but I saw red. I couldn't stop thinking about it all day. I hated myself. I shouldn't have snapped at her. I wrote in the diary how bad I felt and that I needed to try harder. I knew I wouldn't help the situation by getting irritated. Luckily Alex didn't hold a grudge. But I felt bad about it for a long time.

This was another occasion about learning from my mistakes. I am very lucky to have Alex as my wife. She understands the stress I was under and never held a grudge against me if I lost my composure. Even though she would have been well within her rights to hold a grudge against me on numerous occasions!

We were on a 3-week cycle of chemotherapy. They said the middle week would be the worst for side effects and tiredness, and the immune system would be at its lowest. As we entered that middle week, Alex was going to bed at 7:30pm and felt terrible. Those evenings were lonely.

19 November. Sunday.

Alex is tired. I think this is supposed to be the worst of it though and she is doing great. She said she feels like she has ruined our life. She hasn't. It's changed massively but I am appreciating the focus it has given me on what is important. It's nice to not be drinking alcohol and focusing on healthy eating.

My spots are starting to go down. I've not had so many since puberty! Stress is a cunt of a thing.

Throughout all of this period I was practising mindfulness through various podcast and playlists. I think the ability to remain grateful for what we had, rather than focusing on the negative things, really helped at this point. It was important for me to not slip into wishful thinking though. I tried to remain realistic and pragmatic.

I also comment a couple of times about how much Alex is struggling with not being able to do as much as she wants to do. She keeps starting jobs around the house and not finishing them. It's hard because it's difficult to keep on top of the housework at the best of times, but when someone is going around doing half-jobs it makes it even tougher! I didn't tell her to stop though. I know it does her good to stay busy. I just bitched about it in my journal.

The following weekend my sister came to visit with her husband (George) and baby daughter for the weekend. On the Sunday we went to a local farm shop and café.

26 November. Sunday.

I'm tired and grumpy. Go to a farm shop with Rose and George. It's good but I'm pretty snappy with them which isn't fair or nice. I know it too and must not let my tiredness take over.

I've been a bit of a dick these last few days. Need to get to the gym.

It's interesting how many times I acted like a twat whilst knowing I was being one. But it was impossible to stop in the heat of the moment. I hope I wasn't, and am not, a twat at times when I don't realise I'm doing it. It was really hard, especially when I was tired from nights where the girls had been up a lot. I wish I could have controlled it better. It hurt, especially when I was being a knob to people I love and rely on so much for support.

My second paragraph shows how the diary allowed me to keep track of when I was agitated and grumpy. It is pretty easy to spot the correlation between a lack of workouts and me-time, and feeling low.

27 November. Monday.

I asked Alex if I could pop to the gym after going into the office. She said yes but called me after 20 minutes and it's a disaster. I shouldn't leave her with girls on her own it's not fair. She won't ever tell me not to do something she knows I want to do, and she never admits she needs help until it is too late!

Alex is a great wife, and I love everything about her. But man is it annoying that she is just like me and struggles to ask for help. This was a good lesson for me. I knew I needed to blow off some steam but wasn't savvy enough to find a time to do it that worked for everybody else.

29 November. Wednesday.

Meeting with the doctor at hospital. The lump seems to have grown when it shouldn't have. Means the chemotherapy might not be working. I stayed confident and told Alex it wasn't a comparable measurement because the first measurement was from a CT scan and the one from today was with callipers.

It's so shit physically going into the Macmillan Centre. It forces you to accept the reality and severity of it all.

The journey is a continual battering of good news, bad news, no news, and waiting for news. You learn to deal with it but the physical action of going into the oncology department is always rubbish.

The next few days saw my anger rising. It was almost certainly linked to being unable to go to the gym or do anything on my own. I got angry at Alex, with the girls, with my family, with friends, with life. Once again, I knew I was emotional and angry but couldn't stop it or do anything to make it better. It made talking to people harder. It made everything harder. Christmas was creeping up on us. I was hoping for some kind of respite over the festive period.

Annoyingly, it got worse.

3 December. Sunday.

Holy shit. I want to ask for help but literally have nobody to ask. Sophie has a sickness bug and is throwing up constantly in her bed. I don't have any clean bedding left. Oscar (the dog) *is being a cunt and for the first time ever bit me! Charlotte is only a baby and it's so hard to give her what she needs, and Alex is SO tired but won't rest because she knows I need help. I wish she would let me struggle but she knows I'm really struggling right now. My mate from work died this week. Fuck my life! When you're going through hell keep on going and all that.*

The next day Alex got D&V, I threw up, Sophie got worse, and Charlotte stopped eating. My mum was due to come and help at the weekend but tested positive for COVID-19 so had to stay at home. She was coming so I could go and watch the mighty Wimbledon FC with my mate and have a bit of a break; that got cancelled.

Oscar bit me when Alex, Sophie, and Charlotte were all screaming about something. I had grabbed him by the collar to get him out of the way and he instinctively snapped at my hand. It was my fault; he had done nothing wrong and wasn't part of the problem. It was a highly stressful situation, and I should have dealt with it better. He's been my best friend for eight years and it was interesting to see how bad we both felt about it afterwards! He knew he'd messed up and couldn't stop trying to lick and cuddle me afterwards.

The next four days were easily the lowest and hardest of my life up to that point. But we got through it. As the girls started to improve, Alex took a turn for the worse. They found blood and protein in her urine and she had a low white blood cell count. Her chemotherapy was delayed until she was stronger. Delaying treatment is hard to deal with psychologically, but she coped with the setback incredibly well.

Sophie went back to school for the final week before Christmas. It was nice for her, but my diary is full of comments about how hard being a solo-parent is. At one point I went to watch her school carol concert in a lovely old church. It was really hard to keep my shit together. I could have easily started crying my eyes out. All I could think about was how crap it would be if that was what it was like every Christmas. Sat by myself surrounded by happy families.

14 December. Thursday.

Tonight I'm lying in bed just thinking again. Did it last night too. Can't really sleep. Keep thinking about what might happen. What I might do. I need to be a better dad to Sophie. She needs me now.

I was, and still am, focused on the girls. I knew that they would live with the consequences of what was happening for longer than anyone else.

Once again, I learnt from what I was writing in the diary and did something about it. I decided to do something about not sleeping so stopped drinking coffee after midday. It did the trick and soon my sleep patterns were back to normal. It may have been a placebo effect, but

I'm a big believer in action over inaction and perhaps just the fact I was actively trying to solve the problem meant my body let me sleep.

Life kept giving us lemons. Alex's Grandad died the next day. She dealt with it amazingly but couldn't make it to funeral. Everyone said they understood but I felt so sad for her.

It was also around this time that we started to really understand the side effects of chemotherapy. The side effects are easier to understand once you appreciate how chemotherapy works. In short, it attacks and kills cancer cells. It does this by finding and attacking fast-growing cells. The problem is that our bodies are full of fast-growing cells that aren't cancer. People go bald because hair is fast-growing. Skin and nails go dry and weird because they're fast growing-cells too. And, of course, our digestive systems are full of fast-growing cells…

16 December. Saturday.

It's beginning to feel a lot like Christmas! Started to decorate the house today.

Set up the tree and all the bits in the lounge. Really pleased with it all. I took the biggest, longest, breath in through my nose and said to Alex "I love the smell of Christmas!".

But after a second or two I realised I wasn't getting the sweet smell of festive pine... I had just sucked in the most horrific, putrid, foul-smelling flatulence you can imagine.

Fucking chemotherapy. So shit. Even ruined putting up the Christmas decorations.

Alex found it hilarious.

We had a good laugh about it, but it stank. As the chemotherapy side effects were starting to kick-in we realised Alex was one of the lucky ones and probably wouldn't lose her hair! This was great for her own self-esteem, but also meant she didn't look like an alien for the girls. This was thanks to the fact she had been offered the use of a cold-cap. It's like a scrumcap that pumps freezing cold gel around your head during treatments. It doesn't work for everyone, but if it does work then it slows or prevents hair loss. I think the cold-cap is great, not only because of what it does but because of what it implies. If we have scientists focusing on keeping people looking good during their cancer treatment, then the treatment itself must be incredible!

20 December. Wednesday.

Fuck. Another appointment with the doctor and the tumour has definitely grown. I'm so sad and angry and scared. On the drive back home, Alex said she was scared. I'm sad about it. We could do with some good news. I've started telling her everything will be OK. I hope it will be.

Going through the treatment was hard. Having the treatment delayed was hard. But being told it's not having the effect it should have been was even harder. It's all well and good staying confident and positive. But when you get given the facts, and they're shit, it really sucks. I found myself being quieter than my usual self. I was very thoughtful about what I was saying. I didn't want the girls to cotton-on to the bad news, didn't want sympathy from friends or family, and didn't want to risk an argument with Alex.

Christmas was great though. We stayed with family for a week. It was awesome having extra people to help entertain the girls. Alex and I got some time together which was precious. She made me laugh so much. But she also cried a lot and needed lots of rest.

27 December. Wednesday.

We drove back last night. Spent the day chilling at home. Everyone tired but we got the house in order. Back to the grind. Alex tired again. I'm tired too now. I'm a little sad. Feel like I've got nobody to talk to around here. Most of the lads who usually text me haven't for a while but it's Christmas so they'll be busy.

After a great week away with lots of help from family it was a bit of a come-down getting home. *Back to the grind.* Sums it up pretty nicely. It's amazing how dealing with cancer very quickly became routine and a new-normal. I find my comment about mates not texting me interesting. I just checked my messaging history and every time I text someone, they text me back. I'm obviously feeling a little sorry for myself in this entry, but with hindsight I was also guilty of not messaging people over the holidays. I'm certain that if I'd have messaged any of my mates they'd have replied or called. It's a good lesson to learn. Communication is a two-way street. Don't be annoyed at someone for not talking to you if you've not tried to talk to them yourself.

30 December. Saturday.

Alex had round 3 of chemotherapy today. She is not coping well. She is tired and scared and emotional. It's so shit. She is having a go at me a lot too. I know she doesn't mean it. It's because she has a rash and is scared that she has inflammatory breast cancer. If it is this then the outlook is bad. I'm scared too. At one point we both cried and cuddled each other.

Had a cold bath. Apparently they're good for stress. I'm going to do it every day. Managed 5 minutes today.

After the lump continued to grow, they changed the type of chemotherapy drug Alex was on. I remember hoping so much that this one would work. I think the rest at Christmas gave me the strength to get through this bit. I was able to remain calm despite Alex really struggling. It would have been so easy to argue and fall out with each other.

This was also one of the times that showed researching on the internet can be the worst of ideas. We managed to convince ourselves there was a high-likelihood that the rash was something called inflammatory breast cancer. If it was inflammatory breast cancer, the survival odds were rubbish.

2 January. Tuesday.

MRI today. Pretty crap as it's probably grown. Chatted to a young bloke at the MRI whose wife is the same age as Alex. Both said how shit it is. Pretty weird meeting him. Should have got his number. They have two kids who are 9 and 7. This sucks.

Happy new year! This entry is troubling for me to look back on. I'm usually pretty positive about most things and take opportunities when they arise. For me to be so glum about the tumour probably growing and to have not got his number tells me my mind isn't in a good place. I wish I could go back in time and tell myself to be confident about the new type of chemotherapy, and to get this guy's number! I may never have messaged him, but I had a golden opportunity to connect with someone in the same situation as me, and let it slip.

I know some of the cancer charities don't recommend patients buddying up with someone similar to them as the treatment and outcomes can vary massively. But a big part of me wishes I had that guy's number. Chances are our wives will be fine and we could have just sent each other a message every now and then. Or rant to a stranger. It would be like ranting in the diary, but I might get an answer. And if one of us did have a bad outcome then we'd need all the help and support we could get! If you're reading this, mate, I hope you're doing well.

3 January. Thursday.

As expected, the tumour has grown. Possible lump in the armpit too. They may elect to operate sooner than initially planned. Alex sad and scared again. This is crap.

I still sound uncharacteristically negative about the situation. As we've gone along this journey, I've realised that there is always an option and always a plan. If things get worse the system is designed to automatically offer the treatment with the highest chance of success. Medical science is incredible. Even if we got the worst of the worst news and were told the cancer was incurable, there are many treatments that can allow people to live many, many, years relatively normally. And if you think those treatments didn't exist a decade ago, just imagine what will be available in 5, 10, or even 20 years from now.

4 January. Thursday.

Alex is in pain today. Abdominal cramps and painful bones! Relatively common side effects apparently. So shit. She is acting odd too. I think the drugs are playing with her moods. This is crap with kids. Life's hectic and doesn't stop. No time to be with Alex or focus on quality time for us. It's exhausting. I'm doing my best but it's fucking hard.

Bone pain! I didn't even know that was a thing. I remember asking the nurse what it was like and all she could say was your bones hurt. Imagine that! Literally torture. As if everything else isn't bad enough, Alex's bones are now painful!

Re-reading my diary entries over this period is difficult. I notice once again I'm very negative for the fourth or fifth day in a row. I remember this being a dark period. We didn't have much help from friends or family for one reason or another. I could have really done with speaking up and asking for help.

5 *January. Friday.*

Last night was scary. I was dreaming about how hard life is and if I killed myself it would all go away. Woke up and continued to reason with myself that it was a logical thought to be having. Then I caught myself and stopped. I cannot think like that.

What a berk! How on earth did I think dying would help the situation? Literally the last thing anyone needed at that point was for that to happen. I'm proud of myself for stopping the thoughts, but more so for actually writing them in the diary. I have never been, and hopefully never will be, anywhere close to wanting to kill myself. But this shows the effect that days, weeks, and months of stress and sadness can have on a person. Luckily, I remember this was the only time the concept of suicide came into my head. I am grateful for that.

Worryingly though, over the next few days I was in a bad way. I recall being so angry and shouting at Alex and the girls. I felt like I had nobody to talk to. I felt isolated. It continued until the 9th of January.

9 January. Tuesday.

Got to the gym. Made me feel better. I need to train more often. Complete change. Cleared my mind completely. In a much better place.

My mate from uni text me, we haven't spoken in ages. I think she knew about Alex but she pretended not to. Later on, she called me after everyone else had gone to bed. She was really nice. I realised I sounded miserable. She's a good friend. I should talk to more people.

10 January. Thursday.

Got to the gym again. Massive difference. Way more patience. Tidied the house. Feel so much better about myself.

Who says men aren't simple? All I needed was to go for a run and lift some weights and I'm as good as new! Seriously though, I remember this gym session so clearly. I could actually feel the stress leaving my body and the endorphins rushing about. It felt so good. I know it sounds simple but physical wellbeing is so important. Never underestimate the good it can do. But, also never underestimate how hard it can be to make time to do it!

An example of how hard it can be to maintain even the best intentions can be seen with my cold bath idea. You might remember I decided to have a cold bath every day (diary entry 30 December). The physical benefits are numerous, as are the potential benefits for your mental health. I knew physical wellbeing was important and I decided cold baths were something I could easily do at home and fit in around the daily routine. I think I managed four. The idea was good, but I lacked the motivation and perseverance to make it happen.

Casandra (*my mate from uni*) is a great friend. I don't know why I hadn't told her about Alex. But, thinking about it, I didn't actively broadcast the news to anybody. I'm not sure if it was because I was avoiding talking about it, or if I thought people wouldn't be that bothered. I think the main issue was probably my dislike of sympathy. I don't mean I am not sympathetic, I just don't like being on the receiving end of it! I know now that it is better to tell people and be open and honest, but I still hate it when people give me 'that look' or ask in an overly sincere voice 'but how are you?'.

I think it is linked to not wanting to appear vulnerable. By advertising the issue, I would be accepting something was wrong. This was exacerbated by it being an issue I had very little control over. I don't like the feeling of helplessness. I've come to learn, however, that there's often occasions when showing vulnerability and accepting help as an individual will help everyone around me.

14 January. Sunday.

Nice day today. Did nothing but we did it as a family.

I remember these days. It was nice to just be with each other. We didn't try to clean or tidy the house or do any specific activity. It was really nice just to be together.

On the 19 January we had round four of chemotherapy, the second dose of the new drug. I never knew how varied chemotherapy can be. I'd heard about there being stronger, more severe, types but I thought this was just dose size. It turns out that there are loads of different types of drugs that sit under the umbrella-term chemotherapy. They all work slightly differently and have slightly different side effects. In some countries they will test the cancer to see the most effective type of drug to use.

Alex was also given an injection of an antibody drug called Phesgo. Some of the biopsy results had shown it should be effective against her type of tumour. This was her first dose, and she may have to have it periodically for the rest of her life. The syringe was massive! The biggest I've ever seen. The first dose has to be bigger than the follow-on ones. And the nurse just squeezed it all into Alex's thigh. She was, and is, so brave. It looked like a golf ball under her skin by the time it was all in! The bruise lasted for weeks.

20 January. Saturday.

Sophie's 5th birthday! She is amazing. Such a bundle of joy. My mum and dad took Charlotte swimming so me and Alex could spend some quality time with Sophie. We had breakfast in bed (waffles). Then I took Sophie to her gymnastics class followed by lunch at a cafe with my dad. She fell asleep on the way home. Then we made brownies and played libraries. I love her so much. She is brave and great.

It was a low-key birthday but one we all really enjoyed. In the middle of all the rubbish that was going on it was so nice to have a special day together. That evening I remember feeling relieved that we had managed to give her a nice day.

24 January. Wednesday.

The rash is cancer. But the plan is to keep on going with the chemotherapy. The surgery will be big. Feel sick. I said thank you to the doctor who broke the news to us. Everyone says Alex looks amazing. She is beautiful.

The rash coming through the skin was cancer, but wasn't inflammatory breast cancer (as we had convinced ourselves since 30 December). It was cancer cells coming out of the tumour and displaying in the skin above it. This was a welcome relief, and a timely reminder that you can't compare Google with medical school. However, it was still bad news (just not as bad as it could have been). It meant that the surgery was going to bigger than we thought. They would need to remove more of the skin and lymph nodes than initially thought.

28 January. Sunday.

Took Charlotte and Sophie out for coffee and cake at a café. Loads of old people randomly spoke to us and said enjoy these years! It's so sad without Alex.

Had another nosebleed today. Hopefully just scratched it but I think it is stress.

Yet more physical manifestations of stress. I remember trying to kid myself that I must have scratched my nose, but I knew I hadn't. It was just my body's way of trying to tell me something was wrong.

31 January. Wednesday.

Appointment with the plastic surgeon today. He seems very experienced and confident. I'd read somewhere you should ask a surgeon how many operations they have done so you can gauge their competence. He said over 4000.... Lol. I think he is competent. Went out for lunch with Alex to Wagamama's. Felt like the old days.

We had to drive to a different hospital about an hour and a half away to meet the surgeon. It was a full day out and we both really enjoyed it. It's odd how surreal it is. We were taking it all in our stride but it was absolutely not normal.

2 February. Friday.

Today was horrible. Alex tried to do lots and maxed herself out. But she isn't listening to me. I was bathing Charlotte and Sophie needed entertaining, I asked Alex 5 or 6 times to play with her but she was focused on doing something else. Sophie really wanted attention and ended up hitting and spitting at me. Then Alex shouted at both of us. Sophie cried loads and it took me ages to calm her down. Charlotte looked so confused bless her. Alex felt terrible straight away. I need to realise when Alex isn't with it and look after her more.

This was my fault. I kept asking Alex to do something when it was obvious she was in a bad place. She needed me to let her be, and not ask anything of her. For the vast majority of the time Alex coped amazingly. But sometimes we just need a break. On this occasion I was too dumb to realise she needed a break. I felt bad about it for ages too.

5 February. Monday.

Took Alex to clinic. The lump is shrinking!!! Yes yes yes. So very happy. Get in. Chemotherapy is winning. Best news in ages. Was also the first time the doctor spoke to me and not just Alex. It's odd always sitting there like a lemon. They make me sit on the other side of a curtain when they examine her. It's not anything I've not seen before!

And just like that, life got better. It's funny how bad news makes you dread going to appointments. Makes you concentrate on the negatives. Makes staying confident harder and harder. Negativity breeds negativity. One little bit of good news changed all of that. It was such a difference to know for sure that the treatment was working.

I remember feeling shocked when the doctor made small talk with me. Up until this point I may have been asked my name, or to confirm who I was (husband), but that was as far as I was included in 99% of the consultations. It was nice to be recognised as being in the room. I know Alex is the patient and it is rightly all about her. But I am there with her every step of the way.

Alex had her fifth dose of chemotherapy on the 8th of February. The next day I wrote:

9 February. Friday.

Wow Alex has been hit hard this time. It's horrible to see. She is sad and fed up but getting on with it. I love her so much, this is shit. I'm so glad my mum and dad are here to help. I got to go to the gym which was needed and then went on a dog walk with Alex. I'm angry.

Once again, it's clear to see the ups and downs of going through treatment for cancer. We were so high after being told the lump was shrinking. It was shrinking because the chemotherapy was working. The chemotherapy was working because it's fucking strong stuff. Because it's strong stuff it really fucks you up. This made life hard for everyone, not least Alex.

I'd cottoned on the importance of looking after my physical wellbeing by this point and was prioritising it pretty well. I don't mean just going to the gym but also doing things like getting Alex out for a walk. It wasn't a long walk at all, but it got us both outside in the fresh air and gave us time together. I enjoyed those walks even though we often cried.

10 February. Saturday.

Great day on the sofa doing nothing with Alex. Mum and Dad took the girls out all day which gave us some much-needed space. Alex is suffering again and emotional. It's really hard to live with.

We were unlucky that our nearest family live about 4 hours away from us, but lucky that people were willing to visit and help pretty regularly throughout the treatment. I remember this day really well. It was nice to just be the two of us. Not having the girls around was quiet and odd, but meant we actually got to relax and be together without any distractions.

13 February. Tuesday.

Alex is struggling. She has diarrhoea again and now a rash on her arse which is so bad she literally screams! She was crying loads and felt even worse because Sophie saw her. It's really hard. I feel numb at the moment. Really odd.

Living with the side effects of chemotherapy is so tough. It's better than the alternative of not treating the cancer; but they're still really hard to deal with.

The psychological battle of wanting to protect the girls whilst being honest with them was a constant challenge. I think we had been good at not hiding anything, and Sophie understood what was going on most of the time. But nobody wants to see their parents in pain. Especially not a 5-year-old. It's torture imagining what she was thinking about whenever she saw her mummy in pain or me crying.

Later that evening I added this next paragraph to the entry:

This is the hardest fucking thing I have ever done. Charlotte won't fucking sleep again. Fuck my life. How the fuck has it come to this. 35 tomorrow and I have a wife with cancer, a 5-year-old, and a 1-year-old. My friends and family live fucking miles away. Fuck this.

It was my birthday the next day and it sounds like I was pretty fed up. It's another rant in the diary, and I'm glad I could say those words there rather than to Alex, the girls, friends, or family. I was angry and couldn't see all the good things we had. I have great friends and family who will do anything for me. But at that moment I was hurting. Maybe I was just pissed off about turning 35 and being closer to my 40s than my 20s.

On my birthday I took Alex for a CT scan and then to a friend's house for lunch. It was a nice day out and we had cake and laughed about a lot of things. Turning 35 wasn't so bad after all.

The next week was relatively uneventful. By that I mean Alex struggled with stomach cramps, I remained unpredictably angry, Sophie had fun at school, and

Charlotte remained blissfully unaware of what was going on.

20 February. Tuesday.

I am sad and scared again. This sucks. It's the unknown and worry of what might happen that's the worst. It's hard to stay in the moment and appreciate life. I feel sorry for the girls. I hope I am doing a good job.

21 February. Wednesday.

Hospital appointment day. A lot of waiting around. Feels horrible waiting to be seen. Alex is scared. We were finally seen, and it has shrunk again! This time we were a little less joyful. It's hard to be happy. I'm starting to show signs of stress in my body I think. Spots are back and my hair line is receding.

I was feeling pretty low, and the physical manifestations of stress made life even harder. The evidence you're stressed is right in front of you and you can't hide from it.

My imagination didn't help. Just thinking about what might happen made me realise there was a very real chance that Alex could die from this. And then what?

Then I'd have to be a good dad. Otherwise we'd all be fucked.

The difficulty in being happy is interesting too. The ability to be happy and not feel like it's an unwarranted emotion was a real challenge. I remember thinking what was the point in being happy about a shit situation becoming a little less shit. It was easy to become fixated on the finish line and only imagine being happy on the day we got the 'all clear'. Sadly, though, the fact is we will probably never get the 'all clear'. For the rest of Alex's life we will probably have frequent or infrequent check-ups and the dread of waiting for results. She may even be on medication for the rest of her life. It is very difficult to learn how to be happy whilst constantly stressed and worried.

27 February. Tuesday.

Everyone has a cold. Makes it so much harder. Scared about giving it to Alex. Feel like crap. Tired. I'm worried about my mental health. Hopefully I'm not depressed.

We were about four or five months into living with cancer and had a pretty good routine that was manageable to maintain. Apart from when the smallest thing went wrong. Like a simple cold, or a single sleepless night with the girls. These minor things that are part of being a young family made our new-normal life extremely difficult. It's hard to explain how such a minor thing can have such a disproportionate effect on your ability to communicate or do the housework or even remember basic information like a shopping list.

29 February. Thursday.

Sixth round of chemotherapy, and hopefully the last! But Alex is stressed and scared still. She is very irritable and that makes life hard. I've realised in some conversations I just need to listen and not say anything. Hopefully this is the lowest point we get to.

1 March. Friday.

Alex is mad at me all the time and so angry about everything. It's hard because everything I do is wrong and infuriates her. I choose to stay quiet and that makes her more mad! Wish I knew what to say.

I can imagine Alex reading this and laughing at the idea of me ever holding my tongue. I may have realised I needed to just listen, but actually doing it was a different matter. I've spoken a lot about communication already. It is a two-way process, but sometimes it needs to be one-way. Knowing when to shut-the-fuck-up-and-listen is a skill I'm yet to fully master, but I'm working on it.

3 March. Sunday.

Better today but Alex is still struggling. She is scared about the operation and recovery. I hope she knows I will do everything I possibly can for her. I hope she comes through it. Been thinking about if she dies again. Life would be hard.

Understatement of the century. Life would be unbearable! It is amazing where the mind wanders at the oddest of times. Thoughts just bubbled up and I would think about what might happen in the future. How I'd manage with the girls, what I'd to make money, how I'd stay sane! I think it's part of my personality to make contingency plans when I can see bad things potentially happening. I think it is similar to chanting out loud that Alex had cancer. Rehearsing it in my mind allowed me to accept the reality of it all, and if the worst did ever happen, I hope it might soften the blow. In my opinion, it wasn't morbid, or even bad, that I had these thoughts. Acceptance was key for me and helped me process what was happening. I'm not a qualified psychologist though, so maybe it's not good advice for someone else to follow.

7 March. Thursday.

Feeling low again. Charlotte poorly and took her to the doctors. She has tonsilitis. Life is so shit. The girls crying and screaming really gets to me. I don't have the patience for this!

Having young kids is difficult at the best of times. Going through this has increased the respect I have for single parents. I don't know how they do it.

Looking back at the diary extracts, I am upset about how negative they are and how much pain I seem to be in. At the time I was putting so much effort into staying confident for Alex and trying to keep life as normal as possible for the girls that the diary was the only place I would let myself rant. I didn't even really talk to my mates about how much I was struggling or hurting internally.

I took pride in maintaining the façade that I was OK. It made me feel good that I could be a good husband and good dad. I know some people say men are rubbish at talking about emotions and should avoid being the strong silent type. I think being strong and silent was exactly what my family needed. The girls didn't need to see me being angry about the situation, Alex didn't need to know how scared I was about the future. I took pride in how I handled the situation. I spoke to some people about my feelings, but nobody got a full download of where I was at. I'm glad I had the diary to express my negative emotions.

10 March. Sunday.

Mother's Day. I think Alex had a good day. I'm glad my mum helped prepare so many nice things for her.

Grandma saved the day once again. I'm not very good at birthdays, Christmas, or Mother's Day. As an example, one year I kept a list of everything Alex mentioned she wanted in the months leading up to Christmas. I was amazed at her disappointment on Christmas day when she opened a sack full of presents that included flint rollers, shoe deodoriser, and a miniature hot water bottle. Some people are just impossible to please. Anyway, my mum had prepared a load of presents and cards with the girls that went down a treat. We had a great family day and life was good.

12 March. Tuesday.

Feeling pretty good today.

No idea what happened that day but it's nice to see a positive entry.

15 March. Friday.

Pre-Op appointment. Went well. After it we all went to Sophie's school to watch her sports day. So much fun. She has so much confidence and great friends.

This was the end of the Alex's chemotherapy treatment. I'd learnt a lot about the process and the side effects, and was starting to accept the new-normal we were living. It had been really tough on Alex, but she had got through it amazingly well. I realise now how therapeutic keeping the diary had been for me. Sometimes I remember frustration or anger or sadness building and rather than dwell on it or let it build I would start thinking about what I would write in the diary. Writing the emotions down helped me deal with them, keep them to myself, and not make a shitty situation worse. I like to think that outwardly I was happier, more stable, and more positive than probably comes across in this book. Maybe I was, maybe I wasn't. But I am proud of how we all dealt with it.

Surgery

Alex needed two operations. The first one was considered *minor*, but still required a general anaesthetic. They conducted a sentinel node biopsy from the lymph nodes under her armpit. This meant they cut a small hole and took some of the lymph nodes nearest to the tumour. The presence, or level, of cancer cells found in the lymph nodes would dictate the size of the second, *major* surgery.

17 March. Sunday.

Saw Alex's dad and aunt today. It was really nice to interact with adults. But the best thing was that they played with the girls and I watched the FA cup final. Go on United! Loved it.

Had a couple of beers and watched the football. In a great mood. Pretty simple recipe for success. Sure, it wasn't in a pub, or with my mates, but it felt awesome.

19 March. Tuesday.

Pre-Op for Alex but when Molly arrived her son was sick in the car! Poor little lad threw up everywhere. It meant I stayed at home with Charlotte, and Alex went on her own. Feel shitty about that.

Our childminder, Molly, has been exceptional throughout this whole period. She started looking after

Charlotte about 3 months before Alex was diagnosed so has been through it all with us. We've said so many times how lucky we are to have her. We trust her completely and she has been so helpful every time we have needed it. We live a long way away from family, but Molly has more than made up for it. I think anyone going through something similar to this needs to find their Molly.

I'd managed to go to the vast majority of appointments with Alex, except the occasional line-flush or check-up that was deemed routine. I'd have liked to have made it to the pre-op meeting as they can be very overwhelming. Doctors live in a highly specialised and technical world. To a certain extent they dumb some things down for us mere mortals, but generally they bombard you with a plethora of complicated and unusual words to describe what's going on and what they're going to do about it. I tried to make it to every meeting with the doctors so I could try to keep track of what was going on and ask the questions I know Alex may be too maxed-out to ask.

21 March. Thursday.

Alex's last Phesgo. I went with her. The injection looked painful and the room was hot. I knew I was in trouble. Pretty much fainted. For fuck's sake. Twat. I really struggle to see her in pain. And now she will worry about me being in the room for treatments and will try to hide any pain she is in.

I knew I'd have to talk about this day. It is excruciatingly embarrassing. And, even more embarrassingly, I have a history of it. I've never told anybody, but I also fainted when Alex was giving birth to Charlotte. There's something about seeing Alex in pain that I simply cannot deal with. Luckily, this time I managed to stagger out of the room and collapse in a chair before blacking out for a few seconds. This was dramatic, but nothing compared to having the crash-team called to pick me up off the floor in the labour ward.

It is yet another physical manifestation of the stress I was under. I have been in many highly stressful situations with work and have been trained to cope with pressure in a variety of ways. None of that matters when Alex is involved. In some ways I like how much it shows I love her, but I wish it hadn't happened. So very humiliating.

The next day Alex had the first, less-major, operation. I spent the day in hospital with her and my dad had the girls at home. Alex was prioritised to go into theatre first so was ready to go home by mid-afternoon. She seemed physically ok, but I knew the events of the day before meant she would hide any pain or discomfort from me.

This was the first time Alex had an obvious physical limitation that the girls could see. Up until now, and largely thanks to the cold-cap, Alex had looked like 'Mummy'. She could do things like give cuddles and play relatively normally. But this was the first time she had bandages and couldn't lift the girls up. It was a challenge for me. I wanted to look after Alex but had to sort the girls out first. I remember on the first night I had so much to do that it was 8pm before I made Alex dinner. I felt bad about that.

23 March. Sunday.

Good day today with my dad and the girls. Alex is worried though and so am I. It'll be a long 10 days waiting for the results. I hope it is not in the glands, but I think we both know it probably is. Been researching it a lot online.

Ah yes, the waiting game. It was, and always will be, rubbish waiting for results and researching the possible outcomes online. I found the waiting far worse than actually finding out. The anxiety built and built the closer we got to results day. At least, on this occasion, they gave us an appointment to go and get the results. Earlier on in the treatment we were told we would receive a telephone call for some results, but after a few days they changed it to an in-person meeting. As you can imagine, the anxiety went through the roof. Although another time they gave us bad results over the phone. So you never know. Waiting is waiting, and waiting is rubbish.

24 March. Sunday.

Good day out with the girls and my dad. Alex asked me what I think the results will say. I said they didn't matter much as the big operation will still happen regardless. The truth is I'm terrified. I really hope it's not spread / spreading.

This was a good example of being strong and confident in front of Alex, but on the inside I'm hurting. She probably saw straight through it as I'm a terrible liar. But the big operation was going to happen, and the results would dictate just how big it would be. It was going to either be big, or bigger. So, I don't think what I said was wrong.

Towards the end of March I developed a chest infection. Once again, a small illness that would usually be nothing more than a minor irritation made life disproportionately harder. I had a good few rants about feeling depressed and not having any patience with the girls. By the weekend I had got a grip of myself and had a nice time at a friend's house for a BBQ on Easter Sunday.

1 April. Monday.

Better day again. Realised I need purpose and focus. Went to the gym with Alex. It was good. She is amazing!

Alex is amazing. She kept her fitness levels up and worked out throughout chemotherapy and in-between operations. It was rare for us to work out together as one of us would usually look after Charlotte and vice versa. I have no idea what my comment about focus and purpose was about. I am pretty sure my focus was on being dad, and my purpose was getting Alex through her treatment. Obviously I felt like I had a bit more capacity and needed more of a challenge.

3 April. Wednesday.

Another black day. Results came back from the sentinel node biopsy. The lymph nodes have cancer cells and micro metastatic cells. That's bad. Means the operation will be bigger and we will have a full body CT scan afterwards to see if it has spread anywhere. I'm so sad. Fucking terrified now. Poor girls are going through so much. Sophie can tell we had bad news. Need to shower her in love.

I tried to stay confident and tell Alex the operation would be a success and that we were doing everything we needed to, but this was hard to take. I remember feeling really sorry for Sophie after these results. Alex was tearful and I was sad, we made it way too obvious that the news was bad. I know how clever and perceptive Sophie is and should have tried keep us away from her after receiving the bad news. We needed more time to compose ourselves but didn't have it.

It was also another good example of online research fucking with your head. If you read about metastatic cancer, it can be summarised as meaning terminal. However, if you really, really, dig into it, the term metastatic cells is different to metastatic cancer. To the uneducated fool (like me), they are hard to differentiate. When I heard Alex had metastatic cells I practically took it to be a death sentence. It was only by really researching it that I found out metastatic cells, whilst far from ideal, are by no means terminal.

Anyway, the news was bad, the operation would be bigger than we were hoping, and now we had the joy of knowing a CT scan and the excruciating wait for results would follow.

The next day I went to the gym and spent the whole-time doing yoga and listening to a mindfulness podcast. It really helped me process the emotions and psych myself up.

My sister and her husband came to visit again. It was really nice having more help around, but I wasn't in a very good place. Once again, I felt bad about being short tempered and not feeling like my usual self. It's amazing how easy it is to be a dick to those you love the most. Heard a song on the radio with the lyrics "strange words come on out of a grown man's mouth when his mind's broke". Couldn't be more true.

8 April. Monday.

Tough day. Went golfing with Kev and we both cried when speaking about Alex. It's so shit. Tomorrow is the biggest day of Alex's life.

Tomorrow is the big operation. Looking back, Kev wasn't the best person to spend some time with on that day. He can be emotional at the best of times. When Alex first got diagnosed, I had a brew with him and he started crying. I had to console him saying it would be OK. I consoled him! But I am better than him at golf, so it seemed like a good idea to go with someone that would make me look good. I think it was really important to have a few hours of me-time. We knew the coming weeks were going to be tough and this was a really nice opportunity for me to get out on my own.

9 April. Tuesday.

Didn't sleep a wink last night. Worried sick. Got up at 4am to drive Alex to hospital. The girls both woke up and weren't happy which hurt. I managed to stay positive in front of Alex before I had to leave her on the ward. Made her laugh a few times which was nice. Now I'm waiting for the phone call saying I can go and see her. Man I'm sad. This is so shit. Life's hard. Feel lonely. Feel scared. Feel sad. Just want it to end. Sat in my car in the carpark crying my eyes out.

Just went to buy lunch but ended up in the Macmillan centre crying to a stranger. She was good and listened.

It's been 7 hours and nothing yet. They said it would be 4 or 5. Feeling scared. Keep imagining she has died and what I'd do if she has.

Got the call. She is fine. It went well. Thank fuck for that.

That was my longest day. It turned out that the operation had gone really well and had only lasted 4 hours. They were just waiting on porters to take her back to the ward. Fuck My Life, I wish I'd just been told that.

I had naively thought that I could sit on my laptop and do some work whilst waiting for the phone call. I was looking forward to some time on my own. I'd imagined reading my book, having a nice lunch, and maybe listening to a podcast or two. As it turned out, I could have really done with somebody with me. Or to have thought about the emotions I was likely to encounter.

I am so grateful for the lady volunteering at the Macmillan centre. She put me in a quiet corner and let me cry whilst I composed myself. I felt awkward and embarrassed. Not just because I'd dumped a 6 foot, 95kg, emotional wreck on her, but because I didn't really have anything to cry about. Alex was being operated on, sure, but she was being cared for by an incredibly skilful team and the chances of complications with a mastectomy are extremely low. I felt stupid. Anyway, I did have a good cry and remain grateful for being able to do so in relative privacy.

After Alex was wheeled back to the ward I spent a couple hours with her but she was pretty spaced out from the anaesthetic, so conversation was minimal. I helped her to get comfortable for the night and then drove home. It was about a 90-minute drive each way and over the next week I used the time to chat with friends I hadn't really spoken to for a while which was nice.

One of the best stress-relievers I had throughout the bad periods was phone calls with old friends. I am fortunate to have some excellent mates, but unfortunate that I don't live close to any of them. I usually see this as a bad thing, but the physical separation made it easier to talk to them about how I was feeling, vent, or chat about something completely unrelated. My friends never judged me for moaning, or asked prying questions if it was obvious I didn't want to talk about the cancer.

The next day was challenging but good. Alex sat up in bed and was eating food and in good spirits. She had 'drains' in which were crazy to look at. They were literally three tubes coming out of where they operated that drained away the excess fluid to prevent swelling. It meant she carried around a small tote bag with three plastic containers full of bloody-yellowy-clear liquid. Very gross.

10 April. Wednesday.

Day with Alex. It's odd. She is sometimes sad, but generally happy. I find myself focusing on acceptance. Just accept what is happening and deal with it. Live in the moment.

The mindfulness podcasts I had been listening to definitely helped me through the days after the operation. There was no point wishing the situation away and feeling sorry for ourselves. What was happening was happening. Accepting and understanding it made it easier for me. I made sure I listened carefully to everything the nurses and doctors said. Alex was recovering from major surgery; I hope knowing that I was paying really close attention to what the medical staff said allowed her some peace of mind. There was a lot to take in.

It was also important to accept the state of the NHS and understand the need to help the system as much as possible to. It shouldn't surprise anyone to hear that the NHS is constantly in a battle to provide the highest level of care despite numerous obstacles. Without getting too political, we saw this first hand. There were several occasions where Alex or I needed to go hunting for staff to get medication on time or sometimes even check someone was looking at the right notes! This is most certainly not an attack on the staff members we met and worked with. Without exception, they were excellent. The NHS is under-funded and under-resourced, the reason it still functions to an incredibly high level is thanks to its people.

12 April. Friday.

Alex doing amazing. I realised today that there is a chance she now has no cancer in her body. I hope that is true! I know it's unlikely but holy shit it would be great if it's true.

This was a great feeling. It was great when I said it to Alex. I could tell she hadn't considered it that way. I knew she wouldn't let herself believe it too much. But over the next few days I heard her repeating it to other people. I think this was an area of hope or positivity we both really hung on to. The physical action of removing something from her body allowed us to believe that the cancer was being beaten, and would be beaten.

Despite this morale-boost of a thought, the next day was hard following a sleepless night with Charlotte. Sometimes it felt like everything was against me.

13 April. Saturday.

Terrible night with Charlotte. Shattered. She was screaming constantly. I think she is teething. It's hard. There must be so many other people who go through this, and harder, and get no recognition. It's a thankless task!

I realise now how hard caring can, and must, be for some people. They are the ones who deserve recognition and support. I find it sad now when I see news stories about carers struggling to survive with little or no support themselves. It's embarrassing that I had to live through this to feel this way. We need more compassion in the world.

14 April. Sunday.

Alex is coming home! Woweee. Cried on the way to get her. So happy. She is the toughest person I think I've ever met.

Alex called me to say she could go home. It was two days earlier than we expected. She asked me to get her a coffee from the café on my way up to her, and she surprised me in the queue! It was so nice. I'm so proud of her.

16 April. Tuesday.

Sophie started playing up with my mum. It's so hard for her. Both of them I mean. I just hope we are helping Sophie with everything she needs to cope. She will be back at school soon so that should help.

This was difficult to deal with. It was obvious that Sophie's behaviour was her struggling to process her emotions. It must have been hard for her to see Alex return from hospital bandaged, frail, and tired. Sophie would hit and spit and shout over the smallest of things. Luckily, we had read books about how to deal with it. It wasn't easy, but we stayed calm, and I think we did a good job. It was more difficult for my mum who hadn't read the books. I tried to explain to her what she needed to do but I knew she felt bad that she couldn't help as much as she wanted.

It's hard when people want to help but can't, or even sometimes make it worse. Then you have to deal with the emotion of that person being disappointed too! Once again, it comes down to clear communication. I found blunt honesty was the best policy.

I also recalled that one of the parents at school offered to help with childcare and told me to avoid the stereotypical British answer of politely declining. I found myself politely accepting, and then not-so politely never taking them up on the offer. It's interesting how I desperately needed help but somehow wouldn't allow my pride to be dented by admitting it, let alone accepting it.

18 April. Thursday.

Alex was worried about a mole so we went to the GP. He wasn't worried at all. Then we went for a coffee together at a café. It was great to spend time being 'normal'!

Hypochondria set in for both of us at different times and to varying degrees. Alex became obsessed with a particular mole, as did I at one point. Neither turned out to be anything at all. We also researched non-traditional methods of treating or preventing cancer. I think it is quite common for people to look for any way to gain an advantage over the disease. We read some books and I watched a show on Netflix about reducing the amount of ultra-processed food in your diet. It is more expensive than a 'regular' diet, but I have actually noticed a significant difference since changing my eating habits and reducing my alcohol intake. I must admit that I still occasionally binge on pretzels, crisps and beer when watching sport or have had a particularly tough day or week, but I see this infrequent blip as being good for my soul, even if it is bad for my body.

21 April. Sunday.

I'd like to give something back, or for something good to come out of this. Maybe I should set up an Instagram account and share this (shit) story. Open myself up for conversations with other scared dads.

I suppose this was the day that the idea of turning my diary into a book started. I was, and am, so appreciative of all the help and support we have received. I am also acutely aware that I have been fortunate to have received excellent training in resilience and dealing with adversity thanks to my job. I know there must be many others who haven't had that training. I dread to think how I'd have coped without it.

The very next day I chatted with a bloke who hadn't had my training, but was facing the same, if not tougher, challenges that I was. I hope that by sharing my emotions and journey that I can encourage people in a similar situation to allow themselves to be vulnerable when the situation allows, whilst remaining strong for those who need them to be strong.

22 April. Monday.

Took Alex for a physio appointment. Sat with a 57-year-old bloke whose wife had the same operation as Alex. He's had it rough. He cared for his dad for 3 ½ years before he died. His mate has cancer in his armpit. His colleague died from cancer over Christmas. His parents-in-law need caring for every weekend. He needs to take unpaid time off work to do it all. Tough. And he is in physical pain himself from various things. He is holding it together amazingly. Everyone is fighting a battle you can't see.

Everyone will fight an invisible war with daily battles at some point in their life. The least we can do is help each other every now and then.

Two days later we would get the pathology results of the tumour and tissue they removed during the operation. There were two possible outcomes. It could be great news and look like we were well on the way to curing Alex, or it could be more aggressive than we thought and look like it was spreading. Either way I knew they would give us the news and already have the treatment plan mapped out. It meant waiting though, and the inevitable and increasing dread.

24 April. Wednesday.

(Written in the waiting room) *The wait for the meeting with the doctor is horrific. Feel sick. I'm snappy. Just in a bad mood. Scared it'll be bad news.*

(Written after the appointment) *It was good news! The tumour was destroyed. It wasn't perfect, as there was still a small amount of cancer in the lymph nodes, but it was good news!*

It was odd getting more 'good' news. The next few days were difficult for me. I was feeling tired and fed up, and generally angry again.

28 April. Sunday.

It's been a good day, but for some reason I'm still stressed. We had good news, but it doesn't feel like it. Alex isn't convinced and now I'm struggling to stay calm. I know it is fatigue and a culmination of everything but it's so hard. Don't want to snap.

After Alex's operation she couldn't lift anything for 12 weeks. This meant she couldn't be left alone with Charlotte. This significantly increased my workload. The time I had available for going to the gym, reading a book, or doing anything on my own was drastically reduced. This increased the pressure on me and removed a lot of the things I'd been doing to relieve that pressure. I certainly felt the fatigue slowly building. It was hard.

My mum stayed with us after the operation and had been invaluable in helping with the girls and doing housework. But she had her own life to live and had to go back home after 3 weeks. The day after she left, I made a big mistake:

30 April. Tuesday.

For some reason I went to the gym and did legs. Not done them in ages. Already hurt.

What a stupid, stupid, decision. The Delayed Onset of Muscle Soreness (DOMS) was horrific. I was alone looking after Alex and the girls and now I could barely walk. Sure, it felt good doing a hard workout, but I regretted it for the next 4 or 5 days. Top tip: physical activity is good for mental health, but DOMS is certainly not.

1 May. Wednesday.

Had to pick Sophie up from school as she is poorly. FML. Why can't life just be easy. Cleaned the house and cooked for everyone again. Being a full-time dad is good, but I struggle. Need other things in my life. Miss work. I am irritable and angry.

I was having a bad day and lost sight of how fortunate I was to have an employer who supported me so much; I'd been given 4 weeks off following Alex's surgery. I know now that wanting to go back to work was just craving an escape. Obviously, I would rather spend time at home with my family (*and* be paid for it). But I remember vividly the feeling of wanting to go back to work. For the distraction. To use my brain for something other than childcare or moral support. My frustrations continued over the next few days:

4 May. Saturday.

I'm not thinking clearly. I'm mad. I'm angry. I'm short tempered. I know I am, but I can't stop it. I need to slow down and accept where I'm at. Control what I can control.

I was using the diary to vent my anger again. I don't remember these feelings being shown outwardly at the time. I think I did a pretty good job at keeping them under control.

My training from work was kicking in again: *Control what I can control.* I remember one day Alex was sad because she was wishing she had gone to get the lump checked out earlier. It was making her sad. But that was done. Literally nothing we could do would change what had happened. All we could do was focus on the now. Focus on the treatment. Hopefully this book might raise awareness and encourage people to check symptoms sooner than they might have done without reading it. If you're concerned, get checked. You have nothing to lose and everything to gain.

Worryingly the next night I sat up drinking whisky watching TV on my own. This was the first time I'd had a drink in ages. It felt good. Maybe I liked the idea of being slightly reckless or self-destructive, or maybe I just needed to escape reality a little. I'm sure a psychologist would have a field day explaining why I decided to sit on my own sipping scotch watching 8 Out of 10 Cats Does Countdown. Anyway, it made me feel good. Luckily this was a one-off. I can easily imagine using alcohol as a crutch. To feel lightheaded, to release some emotion, to pass out. I count myself lucky that I know the damage would not be worth the pleasure so haven't fallen into that trap. I reckon there are many people who do. There's loads of help out there if you need it.

6 May. Monday.

A chilled day. I wish cancer hadn't happened to us, but it has. It has put everything into perspective. I've realised I want to be happy with my life in the present and not focused on long-term goals like retirement or crap like that. Live for the now. Enjoy the moment. It won't be like this forever and could become really-really shit really-really quickly.

7 May. Tuesday.

Another trip to the hospital. I'm so stressed and have loads of spots again. They're in a line on my chin. CT scan for Alex to check if there are any other growths in her body.

I've said it before, but stress really does suck. And a physical reminder of it on your face makes it worse. At least I recognised I was stressed. I was becoming relatively good at making sure I ate well and exercised every day to try and deal with the problem.

8 May. Wednesday.

CT Results showed no more tumours! Enlarged lymph nodes but no growths anywhere! It's great news. Alex won't let herself get too excited. I wonder if she will ever believe it has gone.

The results were fantastic news and continued the positive trend we had started to find ourselves on. It was so refreshing. Especially after the string of negative results we had in the early days. Alex told me off at one point for being too happy about the results. She was terrified of being lulled into a false sense of optimism.

We had some interesting chats about telling people about the good news. We had realised that people like to grab hold of good news and take it to mean everything is fine.

On this occasion we noticed that people took a clear CT result to mean Alex no longer had cancer. Whilst this was hopefully true, we knew that we faced a month of radiotherapy followed by further treatments yet to be decided. We were a long way from being out of the woods and it was a funny emotion to be annoyed with people acting as if Alex had beaten it. I guess people are desperate for good news and just want to hear the all-clear. It was good news, but we did have a long way to go.

10 May. Friday.

The pressure of cooking, cleaning, washing the girls, changing the bedding, working, walking the dog, cutting the grass, sorting the finances, tidying the toys, etc. etc. it all adds up and it's exhausting. Made a curry for everyone for tea and poured myself a beer. Alex made a comment about me being the only one who can drive. Literally just wanted a beer and she made me feel bad about it. In that moment I was so angry with her.

But she was right, and I knew it. I also knew I was overreacting. My anger was with the situation we were in, not at her. Luckily, I didn't react and cause an argument. It's interesting how many of these potential flash points there were. They gradually increased in frequency over time and correlated directly with our levels of stress and tiredness. I have relatively good coping mechanisms and could usually prevent myself from overreacting, but nobody is perfect, and I can think of many times when I wish I'd had more self-control. I'm not an expert but the only reason I think I am good at it is because I've been bad at it. Whenever I have overreacted or said something I wish I hadn't, I've found myself thinking about it in excruciating detail and figured out what I could, and should, have done better. Learning from mistakes, and not holding grudges against loved ones who make similar ones, helped me get through the bad times.

12 May. Sunday.

Hot day today. Decided to call my mate I've not spoken to in ages. I find I make excuses for not calling people. Called him even though Charlotte stole half the conversation. Was great to catch up.

13 May. Monday.

Made time for myself to go to the golf driving range and to the gym. Felt great. Needed it.

I knew I was in a bit of a bad place and needed someone to talk to, and to spend some time on my own. I personally find it easier to go to the gym or golf rather than talk to someone on the phone, but I definitely feel better after speaking to someone. I'm terrible at picking up the phone and calling or messaging someone out of the blue. But I've never had someone say they're too busy or tell me I'm being weak and to get on with life. They've always listened or given me good advice or made me laugh or smile. I use my phone for so many things, but not what it was actually designed for – calling people!

The following couple of weeks included some nice family time and a day out with Alex's dad for his 60th birthday. This was a nice period of time as Alex was beginning to recover from the operation. We were spending some really good quality time as a family. Alex spoke to her work and started a phased return, and I spent a little more time in the office. It was still hard as Alex couldn't lift anything heavy so couldn't be left alone with Charlotte and it certainly felt odd to be getting some form of normality back in our lives.

29 May. Wednesday.

Another day at hospital. This time it's bad(ish) news. Alex will need another course of chemotherapy after the radiotherapy. Lower dose than last time though. This is a fucking rollercoaster. Never get used to it.

That was a rubbish day. We had been feeling like life was getting good and that maybe radiotherapy would be the end of it all. But now we knew that after radiotherapy was complete there would be chemotherapy injections every three weeks for another 10-months. It made the fatigue and exhaustion hard to deal with. I felt stupid to have let myself think we could see the light at the end of the tunnel. We still had a very long way to go. Alex needed the chemotherapy because the pathology report from the operation showed the tumour was a more aggressive type than previously thought. The doctor explained the treatment was precautionary and would minimise the chances of the cancer coming back, rather than fighting any cancer they knew was there. This was reassuring but didn't change the fact the finish line had been pushed back about a year.

The news was bad, but at the same meeting we did get confirmation of the dates for radiotherapy, which was good as they had been delayed due to NHS capacity. Alex wasn't fully recovered from the operation but was steadily improving. It felt like the operation was in the past, and we started to focus solely on the next step, radiotherapy.

Radiotherapy

1 June. Saturday.

Took Charlotte swimming and then got my hair cut. Pretty easy to tell the hairdresser Alex has (had) cancer. It's so normal now.

This triggered a conversation between Alex and me. It didn't seem right to use the phrase *Alex has cancer*. Telling people Alex had cancer was now a regular occurrence and wasn't too difficult to do (most of the time). But it didn't feel right to keep saying she *had* it. We were trying to be confident that the chemotherapy and surgery had worked, and the following radiotherapy and chemotherapy were purely precautionary. We started to use the phrase 'Alex is being treated for cancer' or words to that effect, and say Alex was 'Diagnosed with cancer last October'. This may seem subtle, but I think it was a major psychological boost to start using vocabulary focused on the fact the cancer was either gone or being treated. Up until this point *Alex had cancer*. Now we were on the winning side.

2 June. Sunday.

Alex's friends came to visit which was nice. Alex found the CT scan results had been uploaded to the patient portal. She is sad and angry as they clearly stated the chemotherapy didn't do a great job. She is scared and angry and upset. Makes me sad and scared too.

Technology is great, but direct access to your medical notes can be a pain in the arse. Especially for the uneducated masses. Doctors are well trained and experienced in how to tell patients what's going on. Access to raw data, coupled with Google and an intrigued mind, can cause anxiety and frustration. My advice to Alex was to listen to what the doctors had told us. They wouldn't lie and had been clear that there had been a strong partial response to the chemotherapy.

8 June. Saturday.

Fatigue is really setting in for us all now. Good news has meant people forget how hard it still is for us.

The second half of a marathon can be downhill, but it's still a long way to run.

Cumulative fatigue is really hard to deal with. I'll never forget the feeling of just generally being tired all the time. I wanted to go to bed at 8 o'clock every night but would force myself to have at least an hour of doing something constructive. I think this was a time that it would have been easy to slip into depression. It's like when you get a cold on the first day of a holiday; your body has been holding it together for so long that when given an inch it takes a mile. We were physically and emotionally worn out, the end was in sight (albeit pushed back), and the conversations we were having were a lot more positive than they had ever been. But we were exhausted and still had to get through radiotherapy and the subsequent treatments. I'm not saying I wish people had helped us out more, far from it. We had, and have, an excellent support network. I just think it's important to let people know how hard it is.

13 June. Thursday.

Fucking hell Alex is stressed and worried. The delay in radiotherapy is not good for her mental health. She's manic at times, tearful at others. Her mind is mush. She regularly loses her temper. Now it's not just dealing with the treatment, it's knowing it's delayed too. Torture.

It really was torture. I should explain that Alex was scheduled for radiotherapy about 5 weeks later than the official NHS guidelines recommend (another example of data, Google, and an inquisitive mind causing trouble). It's been in the news recently how delays in cancer care are common. Luckily this was the first delay we had suffered. Up until this point it seemed like all the scans, chemotherapy, surgeries, biopsies etc. had all happened very swiftly and efficiently. But that good luck wasn't with us now.

There are probably terms psychologists would use to explain the phenomenon, but in simple words Alex knew she had a life-threatening illness, knew there was medicine available that she needed, but had to wait because of issues outside of her control. I reminded Alex that we had been fortunate up until this point to receive the care we had. The medical staff had been faultless. It was easy for me to say this though, I wasn't the one with cancer.

14 June. Friday.

Numb. Just don't really feel any emotion at the moment. On autopilot.

It was an odd sensation. I think I had become so acclimatised to our 'new-normal' that I'd lost the ability to think clearly. I hadn't cried or had any strong emotions for quite a while and think I was probably a little overly blasé about it all. The feeling of numbness stayed with me for a quite a while. I didn't feel very close to Alex. Maybe this was because we were spending so little quality time together. Alex would often go to bed a lot earlier than me, and we had been sleeping in separate beds so she could have undisturbed nights. I remember thinking I didn't like the feeling and would need to do something about it. I decided the key was to find ways for Alex and me to spend more time together.

17 June. Monday.

Constantly tired. Just have no energy for anything. Realised I've not really laughed or had fun in ages.

20 June. Thursday.

This isn't fair but it is happening.

I was blatantly pretty low. We were in a steady routine, the outlook was positive, and Alex was slowly able to help more with childcare. But somehow this was a really difficult time for me. I think I had grown accustomed to not socialising very much and not spending any time doing things just for me and feeling guilty if I thought I was being selfish. I was struggling to enjoy nearly everything. It probably links back to the pressure being released a little following the news that a positive outcome was now highly likely. I find it very strange that I was this depressed despite knowing we were probably through the hardest part.

21 June. Friday.

Got home and Alex was furious. She had spoken to her work and HR wouldn't follow the recommendations of Occupational Health. She is mad! Crying. Livid. With me!!

This was a rubbish evening. Alex was mad with rage. She struggled to understand why I wasn't mad too. But in my opinion both our employers had been exceptional, for which I will be eternally grateful. I was given all the time and space I needed to support her and the girls, and her direct managers were also very supportive and understanding. We couldn't have asked for more. I am sure that many other people will not be as fortunate as we were. I remember trying to explain to Alex that if the cost of the support we had received so far was just this issue, then that was a price well worth paying. Pick your battles. I like to think that this was a great example of the perspective this ordeal has given me. By stepping back and seeing the bigger the picture, there really wasn't much point in getting annoyed at someone in HR doing their job, probably correctly, and having the rubbish task of telling a cancer patient the procedures they have to follow.

24 June. Monday.

Really fed up today. The weather is hot and everyone is aggy. There's not a lot of joy in my life. Alex getting more anxious about the radiotherapy.

Alex gradually became increasingly nervous about radiotherapy. She could remember vividly how tired and poorly she was on chemotherapy and was dreading it having a similar effect. Even if it wasn't as bad, the thought of being constantly tired and dealing with the inevitable side effects was weighing heavily on her mind. I tried to reassure her, but I was also dreading it. And as you can see from the previous extracts, I'd been in a relatively low place for the last few days and weeks. My morale was dented and energy levels low. But I stayed confident and told her whatever happened, we would manage and cope with it. I reminded her that the radiotherapy was only going to last 3 weeks, and we had support from Molly and my parents arranged to help us.

27 June. Thursday.

First day of radiotherapy. Molly's car failed an MOT so she couldn't come and look after Charlotte! We came up with a plan for Sophie to have breakfast at a friend's house and we dropped

Charlotte at Molly's house on the way to the hospital.

Radiotherapy went well and all the staff are lovely, again.

When we got home Alex cried a lot though. She feels tired and worn out already. I gave her a cuddle.

Life tests you! It was very stressful when Molly messaged to say she didn't have a car. But after taking a moment to think about the problem we quickly came up with a solution. It wasn't that big a deal at all. But it certainly added stress and we could have done without it. I don't think it was the treatment that made Alex tired, but the emotions of waiting and finally receiving the radiotherapy. Anyway, day one was done and all-in-all it had been a success.

30 June. Sunday.

Did a kid swap with our friends. They had our two whilst me and Alex went on a bike ride, then I had their 3 for the afternoon whilst they went out.

Was a great day. Alex cycled 25 miles! She did fantastically! Stopped for a coffee and a cake which was nice.

Alex always amazes me. Two days into radiotherapy and she asks to go on a 25-mile bike ride! She is a superstar. It was an awesome day. It was so nice spending quality time together, and then having five kids running around the house and garden was a lot of fun too. It was a really healthy dose of normality. It did me, Alex, and the girls the world of good.

2 July. Tuesday.

Spoke to Rose on FaceTime. She asked me how I was. I pretty much ignored it. I haven't spoken to anyone about how I feel for quite a while. I'm very good at avoiding the question now.

Alex set off for day 4 of radiotherapy but had a call on the way to say the machine was broken. She was very upset by this.

Two big things to unpack here. Firstly, Alex was not just upset about the machine being broken but more so because she had been told the week before that radiotherapy only works with a minimum of two consecutive doses. She was receiving treatment every weekday for 3 weeks. Missing a Tuesday meant she believed the treatment from the day before (Monday) was not going to have worked because it was in isolation. The nurse told her not to worry and that an extra day would be added to the end of the treatment, but she still felt terrible about it.

Secondly, I had become good at ignoring the question when people asked how I was. I think I was pretty good at ignoring it even before Alex got ill (*classic strong-silent type*). But I'd become a pro by now. I think there's a lot of media coverage about the issues surrounding male mental health, and I know the importance of openly accepting and talking about emotions. But the male role models in my life do not openly talk about emotions very often or in great detail. I don't see this as a bad thing. I am an advocate of people being strong when they need to be strong. Being able to act as a sponge, soaking up other people's sadness and worry, is a good trait in my opinion. As is being able to put on a façade of normality to help others cope with adversity, especially children.

I suppose I don't see the value in being brutally honest every time someone asks me how I am. I'd rather say I'm fine, or make a joke about life being shit, rather than acknowledge the pain I am feeling. Being vulnerable is hard to do, and I prefer to choose the time and place to show my vulnerability rather than display it every time I am asked; how are you?

When you ask someone in my position how they are, expect them to say fine. But understand they're probably not. They'll be working hard at being strong. Help them to be strong, don't force them into showing vulnerability at a time when they don't want to show it. They'll find the right moment that works for them to show it. If you're unfortunate enough to be the person they show their vulnerability to, I'm sorry! Don't worry about what they're saying, they're probably just venting, the best thing to do is just listen.

4 July. Thursday.

Drove Alex to chemotherapy early this morning. I managed to cause an argument in the car. Felt terrible. She screamed that she is dying and can't do anything right. I wish I could fix everything.

The next week was pretty miserable to be honest. I managed to cause a fair few arguments by being a dick. I wasn't in a good way and was struggling to cope. I think the cumulative fatigue was really getting to me. As 'Dad' I was fed up with the pressure and had a general feeling that I wasn't doing a very good job at home or at work. It was a crappy place to be living.

Another thing happened around this time. I mentioned to Louisa, who works on the MacMillan desk at the hospital, that I was thinking about writing this book. She said it was a good idea and gave me a couple of contacts to reach out to. But she did laugh when I called myself a *young* Dad! I guess she has seen many-a-family with parents younger than Alex and me, but it didn't half hurt my feelings. I think I am a *young* Dad; therefore, I am a *young* Dad. But it made me appreciate once again that we are lucky to have the life we have. Sadly, Alex is a lot older than many people who die from cancer. It doesn't make it any easier, but it does help you to be grateful for what we have.

6 July. Saturday.

Listened to a great song today that's going to be my theme tune. Better Man by Keb' Mo'.

It really is a good song:

> Sittin' here in my problem
> What am I gonna do now
> Am I gonna make it
> Someway, somehow
> Maybe I'm not supposed to know
> Maybe I'm supposed to cry
> And if nobody ever knows
> The way I feel, that's all right
> That's okay
> I'm gonna make my world a better place
> I'm gonna keep that smile on my face

> I'm gonna teach myself how to understand
> I'm gonna make myself a better man, yeah
> Climbin' out the window
> Climbin' up the wall
> Is anybody gonna save me
> Or are they gonna let me fall
> Well, I don't really wanna know
> I'll just hold on the best I can
> And if I fall down, I'm gonna get back up
> It'll be alright, it'll be okay

Music plays a big part in my life. I often find a soundtrack for how I'm feeling and enjoy blasting it out whilst driving, dancing in the kitchen, or working out in the gym. It's a nice way to escape reality and let your mind wander. It can be the lyrics, the beat, or having it so loud that it numbs everything else.

11 July. Thursday.

Had sex with Alex. Feel great.

Sex is always fun. Well, it is 99.9% of the time. The only sex I've ever not enjoyed was when we were doing it for the purpose of making a baby. Then it's all about schedules, thermometers, diets, and moon phases. I remember it being pretty rubbish. I mean it was still fun, but not fun-fun. So much pressure, and no spontaneity. Know your job and do it, then get out of the way.

Anyway, it had been a short while since we had last had sex, and we had struggled to spend any quality time together since the radiotherapy had started. On that day we managed to have a couple of hours together without the girls and away from work. It was good to reconnect. I'd love to say we spent the entire two hours shagging, but the majority of the time was spent walking the dog and eating lunch. Sex is obviously, usually, part of a healthy and strong relationship but during cancer treatment it takes a back seat for the obvious reasons. My advice is to try and do it whenever you can. You'll be told by the medical staff when you can't, but if you're not told not to, then do it!

16 July. Tuesday.

Drove Alex to Hospital for radiotherapy and took Sophie with us. It was nice for her to see where Alex goes and for it to be pretty normal. I think she has coped amazingly well with all of this. She is only 5! Last night in the bath she squealed with laughter when Charlotte put a swimming hat on and she said 'she looks like she has cancer"!

Got a place in the London Marathon next year for Macmillan! Need to start training!

By now, cancer had become strangely normal for all of us. It was still really sad at times, but I was probably in the best frame of mind I had been in. I enjoyed being confident enough to take Sophie to the hospital. Both Alex and I had teary and emotional moments every now and then, but I think we had come to terms with our reality, and I was proud of how we were all coping.

I was excited about the place in the marathon. Hopefully I can raise some money for Macmillan. I think I'll spend the rest of my life trying to help the charities who have supported us. This book can help raise awareness and possibly support people going through hard times, and I'll try to do an event every year to raise some funds too.

18 July. Thursday.

Radiotherapy done. It's gone pretty quickly for me, but Alex says it hasn't for her. I'm so proud of her. I love her so much.

After the treatment we had a meeting with the nurses who talked Alex through the next steps. I asked if Alex was now classed as being in remission. They said they don't use phrases like that nowadays. As far as anyone is concerned, she is 'disease free'.

We still have many more preventative treatments to go, and Alex will get periodically checked for the rest of her life. But for now, Alex is disease free. Buzzing.

The next day I started writing this book. I thought it was important to write it while it was fresh and for it not to be tainted by what happens next in life, or for any of the memories to fade.

The End

There isn't a happy or sad ending to this story. Not even an ending really. My intent was to give a raw account of my feelings as we lived through chemotherapy, surgery, and radiotherapy. I believe these are generally the treatments most people will encounter, although all treatment plans differ.

Alex is about to start a treatment of hormone and chemotherapy injections every three weeks for 10-months. I'm not naïve enough to think that will be the end for us. We will deal with whatever happens, and it will become our new-normal.

I'd like to emphasise that this book contains the feelings and thoughts that I largely kept to myself and struggled to talk to others about. I have no doubt that the training I have received throughout my career allowed me to cope and perform relatively well despite the stress and pressure I was under. I know there will be many others who haven't had the training and experiences I have had. To those of you who need some help and advice, I offer the following to pick and choose from:

1. Focus on the children. They will be the ones who live with the impact of this the longest.

2. You can't expect to look after other people if you don't look after yourself.

3. Never forget that communication is a 2-way process.

4. Cry. It helps. But do it on your own terms and don't be ashamed of it.

5. Keep a journal or diary. It's the safest place to vent.

6. It's ok to not be ok. But it's not ok to not do anything about it.

7. Make mistakes, but don't make them twice.

8. Be strong. Be proud of being strong.

If you're struggling with any of the topics I've covered in this book, or with anything I haven't, please don't suffer in silence. There are so many ways to get help. If you don't know what to do, or who to ask for help, then take yourself to your local Macmillan centre and tell them the problem. Failing that, you can always call the Samaritans on 116 123. They will help you.

Acknowledgements

I would like to thank anyone looking, or hoping, for an acknowledgement section. There are many of you who deserve my thanks, and I genuinely mean it when I say: Thank you for supporting me and thank you for helping make this book a reality.

My biggest thanks go to all the doctors, nurses, Macmillan workers, and hospital volunteers we have met along the way. You are all amazing.

All profits from this book will be donated to charity.

If you or anyone you know is able and willing to donate, either as a one-off or on a more regular basis, please scan the following QR code:

Printed in Great Britain
by Amazon